Intermittent Fasting 101

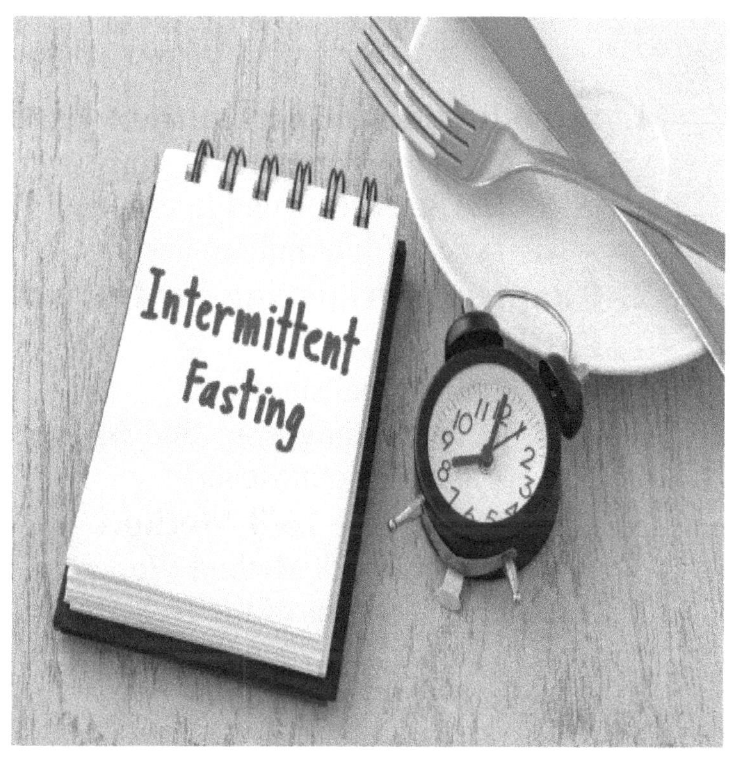

A Beginner's Guide

BILLY SHAM

Table of Contents

(continued from previous page)
   b. Pros and Cons of Alternate Day Fasting
   c. Tips for Success with Alternate Day Fasting

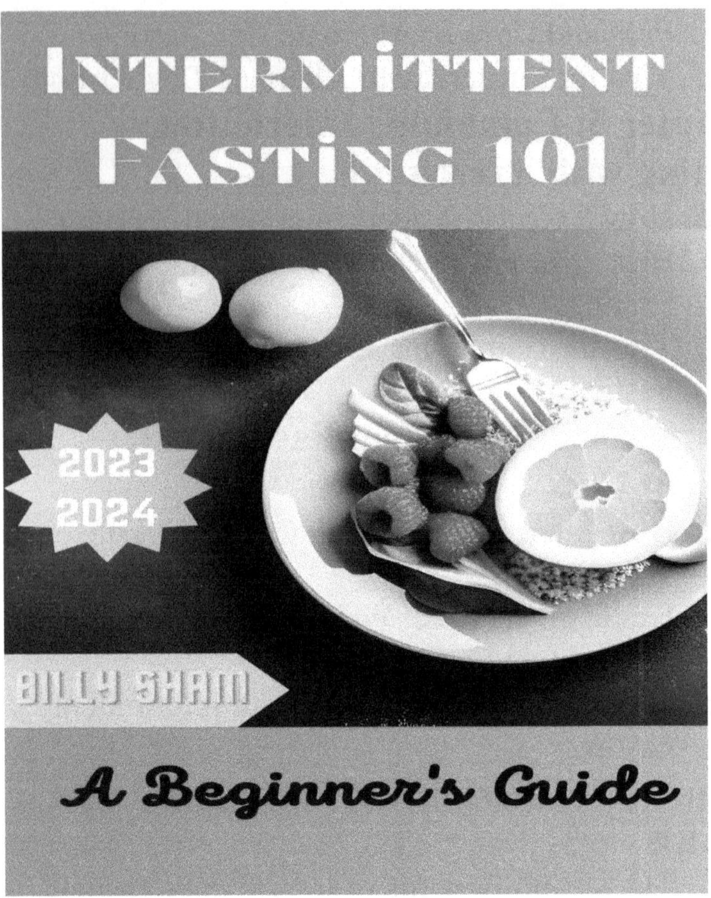

Introduction

Sarah is a woman on a mission. With a passion for health and wellness that runs deep, she has spent years exploring every avenue of healthy living, always searching for the next challenge to push herself further. So when she stumbled upon the book "Intermittent Fasting 101" on the internet, she knew she had found her next adventure.

At first, Sarah was skeptical. She had always been taught that breakfast was the most important meal of the day, and the idea of skipping meals seemed counterintuitive. But as she delved deeper into the world of intermittent fasting, she began to see the incredible benefits that this practice could offer.

For those who are unfamiliar, intermittent fasting involves restricting your eating to specific windows of time throughout the day or week. There are many different methods and protocols to choose from, but the basic idea is to give your body a break from constantly digesting food, allowing it to focus on other important functions like repairing cells and burning fat.

As Sarah began experimenting with different fasting schedules, she was amazed at how quickly her body responded. She had always struggled with stubborn belly fat, but after just a few weeks of intermittent fasting, she noticed a significant decrease in her waistline. Her energy levels soared, and she found herself feeling more focused and alert throughout the day.

But the benefits of intermittent fasting weren't just physical. Sarah also noticed a profound shift in her mental clarity and emotional wellbeing. By giving her body the chance to enter a state of ketosis (where it burns fat for fuel instead of glucose), she found that her mind was sharper and more focused than ever before. And by forcing herself to be more mindful about when and what she ate, she developed a greater sense of discipline and control over her cravings and impulses.

As Sarah's passion for intermittent fasting grew, she began to devour every book, article, and podcast on the subject that she could find. She experimented with different fasting schedules and methods, constantly tweaking and refining her approach to find what worked best for her. And as she shared her experiences with friends and family, she found that she had a gift for explaining the science behind intermittent fasting in a way that was accessible and easy to understand.

Before long, Sarah had become something of a local expert on intermittent fasting. She started hosting workshops and seminars, sharing her insights and expertise with anyone who was curious about this powerful practice. And as word spread, her influence began to reach farther and wider than she ever could have imagined.

Today, Sarah is a respected voice in the world of health and wellness, known for her deep knowledge and expertise in the field of intermittent fasting. She has written countless articles and blog posts on the subject, and her book "Intermittent Fasting 101" has become a go-to resource for anyone who is looking to get started with this practice.

But Sarah's impact goes far beyond her writing and speaking engagements. She is known for her generosity and kindness, always taking the time to answer questions and offer support to those who are struggling with their health. And she is a living example of the power of intermittent fasting, inspiring countless others to take control of their health and transform their lives for the better.

In the end, it's hard not to be impressed by Sarah's incredible journey with intermittent fasting. She has taken a practice that is often misunderstood and demystified, showing how it can be a powerful tool for improving both physical and mental health. And she has done it all with a spirit of generosity, kindness, and passion that is truly inspiring. So if you're ready to take your health to the next level, there's no better guide than Sarah and her incredible journey with intermittent fasting.

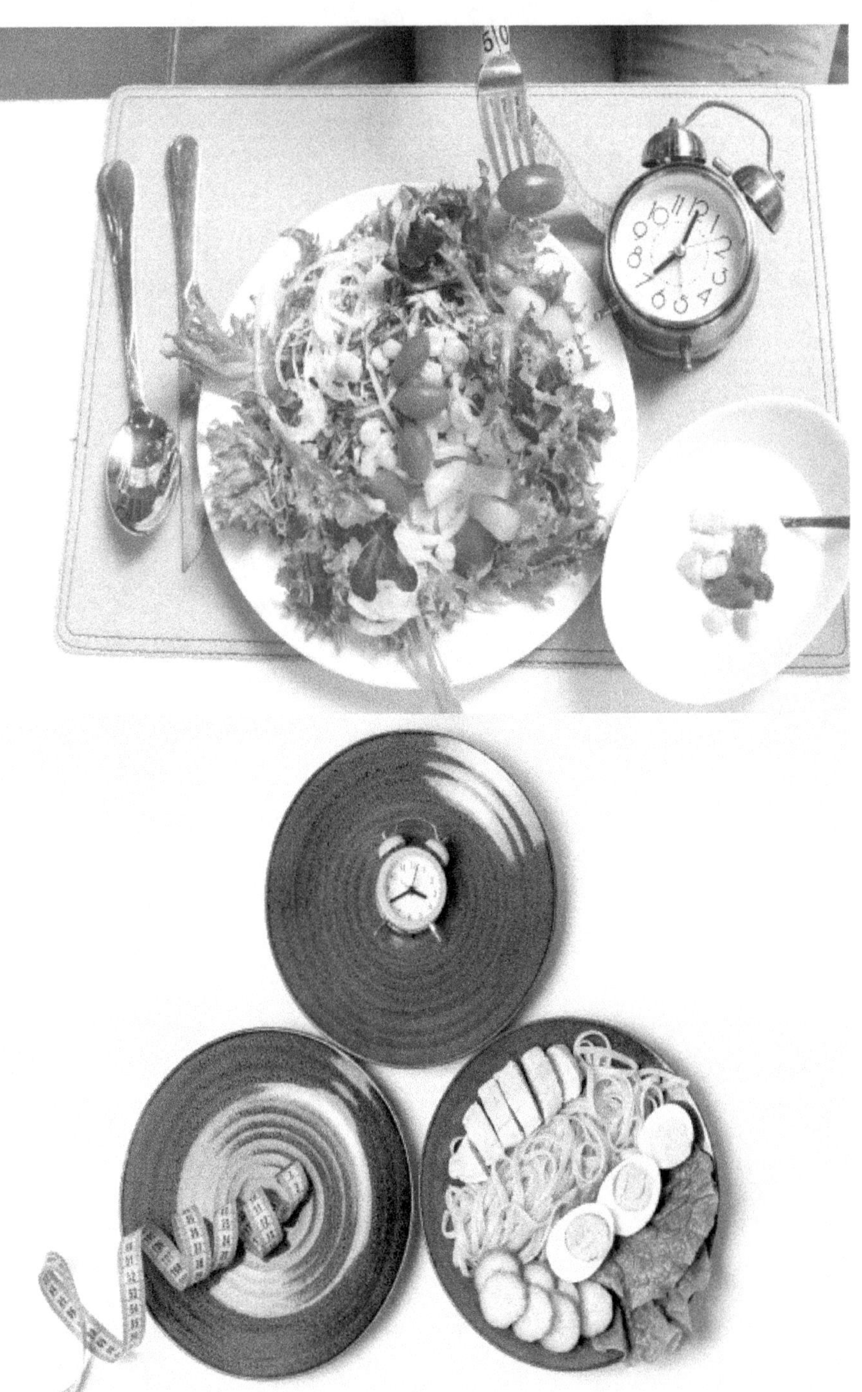

Introduction to Intermittent Fasting

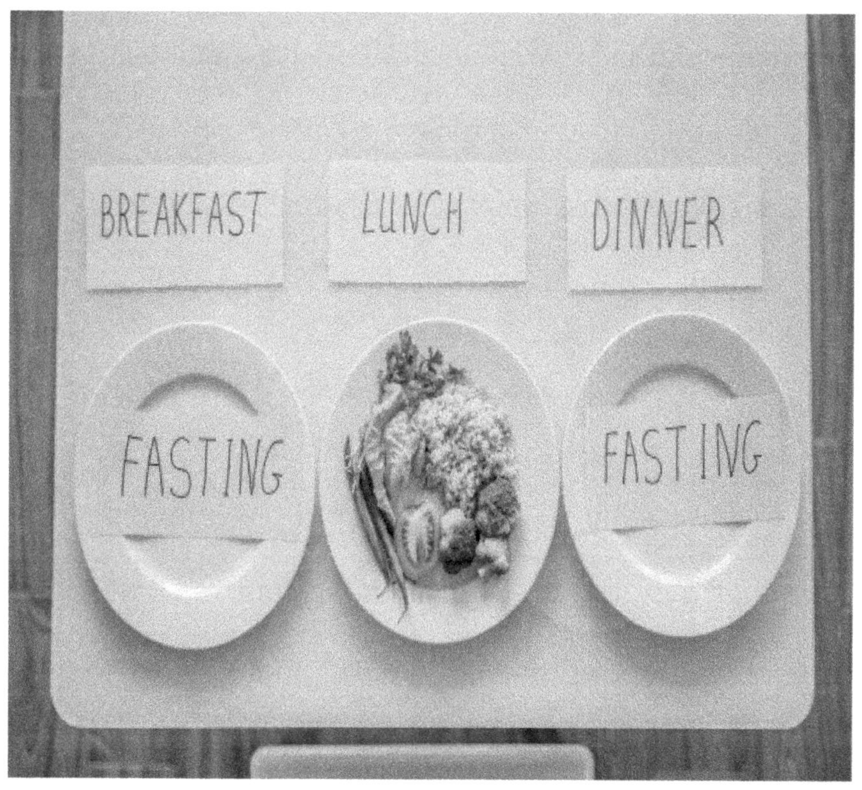

Intermittent fasting is a method of eating that involves alternating periods of eating and not eating, or fasting. It is not a diet in the traditional sense, as it does not involve restriction of specific foods or macronutrients. Instead, it focuses on the timing of meals and the duration of fasting periods.

The concept of intermittent fasting has been around for centuries, but has recently gained popularity as a weight loss and health improvement strategy. Research has shown that intermittent fasting can have a number of benefits, including weight loss, improved insulin sensitivity, reduced inflammation, and improved heart health.

What is Intermittent Fasting?

Intermittent fasting is a method of eating that involves alternating periods of eating and not eating, or fasting. It is not a diet in the traditional sense, as it does not involve restriction of specific foods or macronutrients. Instead, it focuses on the timing of meals and the duration of fasting periods.

The most popular forms of intermittent fasting include the 16/8 method, the 5:2 diet, and alternate day fasting. The 16/8 method involves fasting for 16 hours and eating during an 8 hour window. The 5:2 diet involves eating normally for 5 days and restricting calories to 500-600 for the other 2 days. Alternate day fasting involves a 24 hour fast followed by a 24 hour eating period.

The Science behind Intermittent Fasting

Intermittent fasting works by changing the way the body uses energy. During a fast, the body uses stored glucose (glycogen) for energy. Once glycogen stores are depleted, the body begins to break down fat for energy. This process is called ketosis, and it is associated with weight loss and improved insulin sensitivity.

Intermittent fasting also triggers a process called autophagy, which is the body's way of cleaning out damaged cells and regenerating new ones. Autophagy has been linked to improved brain function, longevity, and disease prevention.

Types of Intermittent Fasting

There are several different types of intermittent fasting, each with its own set of rules and guidelines. Some of the most popular types include:

- **The 16/8 Method:** This method involves fasting for 16 hours and eating during an 8 hour window. For example, eating between 12pm and 8pm and fasting from 8pm to 12pm the next day.
- **The 5:2 Diet:** This method involves eating normally for 5 days and restricting calories to 500-600 for the other 2 non-consecutive days.
- **Alternate Day Fasting:** This method involves a 24 hour fast followed by a 24 hour eating period.
- **The Warrior Diet:** This method involves eating one large meal at night and only small amounts of fruits and vegetables during the day.
- **The Eat-Stop-Eat Method:** This method involves a 24 hour fast, once or twice a week.

It's important to note that not all types of intermittent fasting are suitable for everyone. It's important to consult with a healthcare professional before starting any new eating plan, especially if you have any underlying medical conditions.

Intermittent fasting can be an effective weight loss and health improvement strategy, but it's important to choose the right type of intermittent fasting that is suitable for your lifestyle and health conditions. It's also important to listen to your body and adjust the plan as needed.

It's also important to note that while intermittent fasting can have many benefits, it is not a magic solution for weight loss and health improvement. It should be combined with a healthy diet and regular exercise for best results.

Additionally, it is not recommended for certain populations such as pregnant or breastfeeding women, people with a history of disordered eating, and individuals with certain medical conditions. It's important to consult with a healthcare professional before starting any new eating plan, especially if you have any underlying medical conditions.

In summary, intermittent fasting is a method of eating that involves alternating periods of eating and not eating, or fasting. It is not a diet in the traditional sense and it focuses on the timing of meals and the duration of fasting periods. The most popular forms of intermittent fasting include the 16/8 method, the 5:2 diet, and alternate day fasting. Intermittent fasting has many benefits such as weight loss, improved insulin sensitivity, reduced inflammation, and improved heart health. It's important to consult with a healthcare professional before starting any new eating plan, especially if you have any underlying medical conditions.

Another important aspect to consider when starting intermittent fasting is to ease into it gradually. It's not recommended to start with a very restrictive fasting schedule or to jump into a long fasting period right away. Instead, it's best to start with shorter fasting periods and gradually increase the duration of the fast over time. This will give your body time to adjust and will make it less likely for you to experience negative side effects such as low energy, hunger, or headaches.

It's also important to be mindful of nutrient density during the eating periods. Even though intermittent fasting does not involve restriction of specific foods or macronutrients, it's still important to make sure that you're consuming enough nutrients to support your overall health. Eating a diet that is rich in fruits, vegetables, whole grains, lean proteins, and healthy fats will ensure that you're getting the nutrients your body needs.

Intermittent fasting can also be a great way to improve your relationship with food. By learning to listen to your body's signals of hunger and fullness and by breaking the cycle of constant snacking, you may find that you have a greater sense of control over your eating habits.

In conclusion, Intermittent fasting is a flexible and sustainable approach to health, weight loss and overall well-being. It is important to consult with a healthcare professional before starting any new eating plan, and it's best to ease into it gradually by starting with shorter fasting periods and gradually increasing the duration of the fast over time. Combined with a healthy diet and regular exercise, intermittent fasting can be a powerful tool for improving your overall health and well-being.

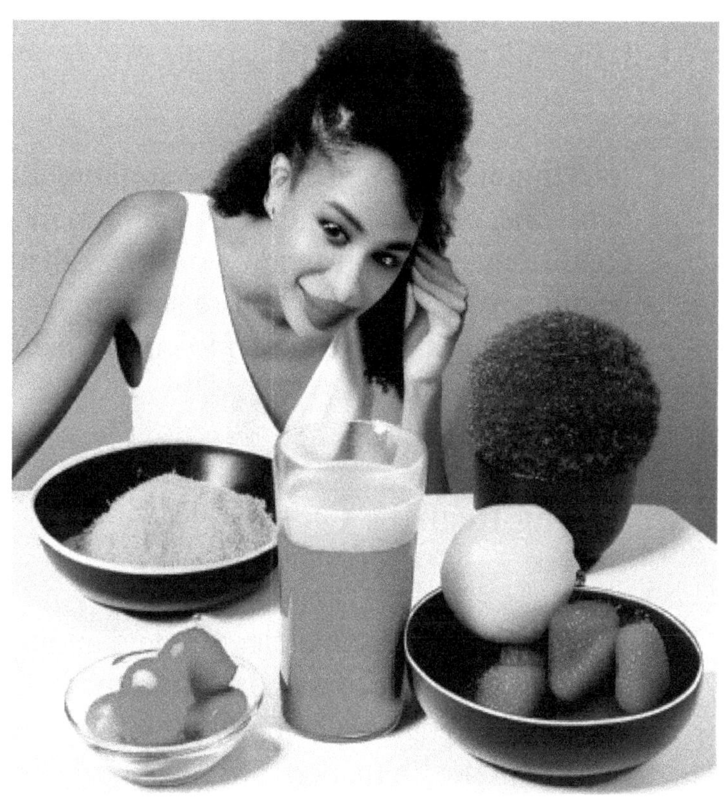

Chapter 1: Preparing for Intermittent Fasting

Intermittent fasting can be an effective tool for weight loss and health improvement, but it's important to prepare properly before starting. In this chapter, we will explore some of the steps you should take to prepare for intermittent fasting.

1. **Consult with a healthcare professional:**

Intermittent fasting may not be suitable for everyone, especially those with certain medical conditions. It's important to consult with a healthcare professional before starting an intermittent fasting regimen to ensure that it's safe for you.

2. **Setting Realistic Goals:**

It's important to have a clear understanding of what you hope to achieve with intermittent fasting and to set realistic goals. Whether your goal is weight loss, improved health markers, or increased energy, it's important to have a plan in place and to track your progress.

3. **Gradually ease into it:**

It's important to ease into intermittent fasting gradually to avoid overwhelming yourself. Start by cutting out snacking or reducing the number of meals you eat, and gradually increase the duration of your fasting periods.

4. Understanding Your Body's Hunger Cues:

Intermittent fasting can be challenging, especially in the beginning. It's important to understand your body's hunger cues and to learn how to manage them. This may involve practicing mindfulness techniques, such as deep breathing or meditation, to help control feelings of hunger.

5. Plan your meals:

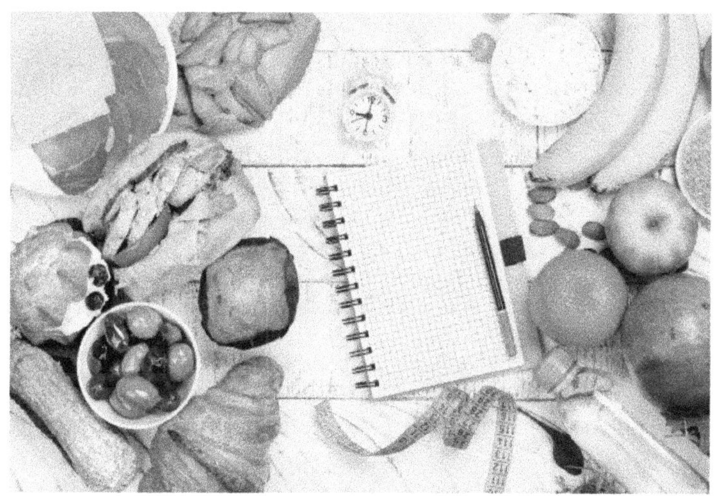

Planning your meals in advance can help you stick to your fasting schedule and ensure that you're getting the nutrients you need. Try to focus on nutrient-dense foods during your eating periods and avoid processed foods and sugary drinks.

6. Meal Prepping:

Another great way to stay on track with your fasting schedule is by meal prepping. This means preparing your meals in advance for the days or weeks ahead. This will help you stay on track with your fasting schedule and ensure that you're getting the nutrients you need.

7. Hydrate:

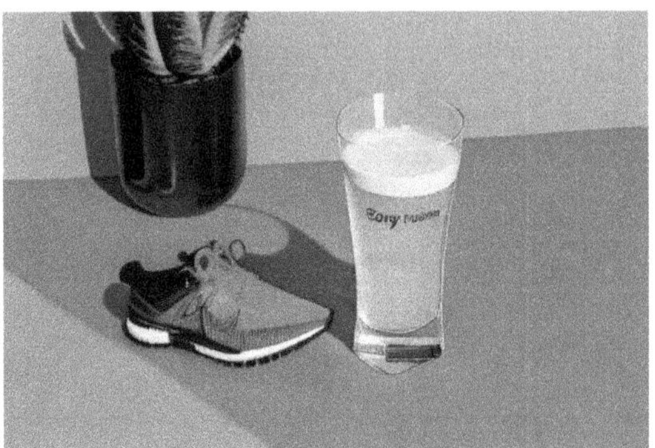

Drinking enough water is essential to maintaining good health, and it's especially important during intermittent fasting. Make sure to drink plenty of water before, during, and after your fasting periods to keep your body hydrated.

8. Stay active:

Regular exercise is an important component of a healthy lifestyle, and it's especially important during intermittent fasting. Exercise can help you stay energized and reduce feelings of hunger.

9. Monitor your progress:

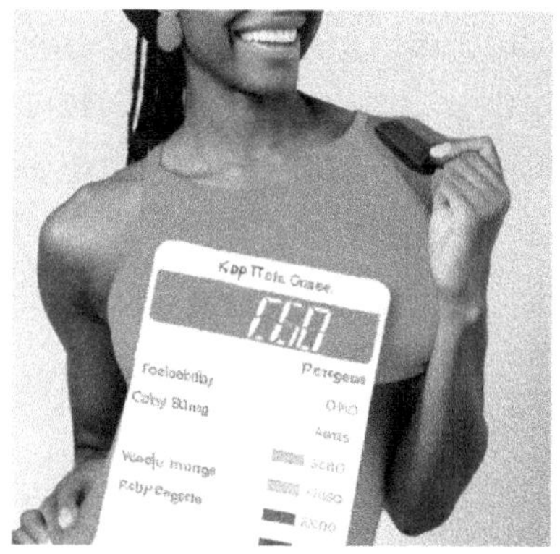

Keep track of your progress by measuring your weight, body fat percentage, and other health markers. This will help you determine whether intermittent fasting is working for you and make any necessary adjustments.

10. **Be patient:**

Intermittent fasting can take time to see results, so it's important to be patient. Keep in mind that it's not a quick fix, but rather a lifestyle change that requires commitment and consistency.

In conclusion, preparing for intermittent fasting is crucial for success. It's important to consult with a healthcare professional, ease into it gradually, plan your meals, stay hydrated, stay active, monitor your progress, and be patient. Remember that it's a lifestyle change that requires commitment and consistency to achieve your goals.

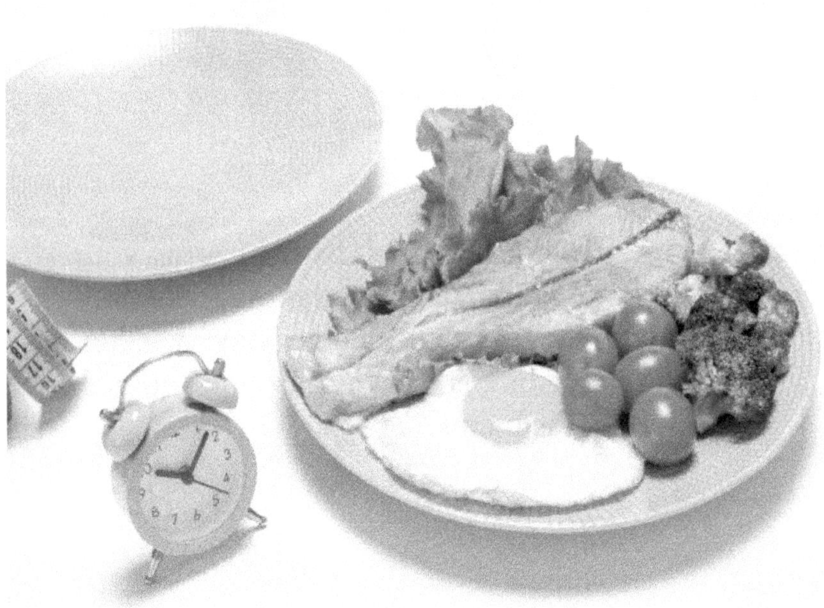

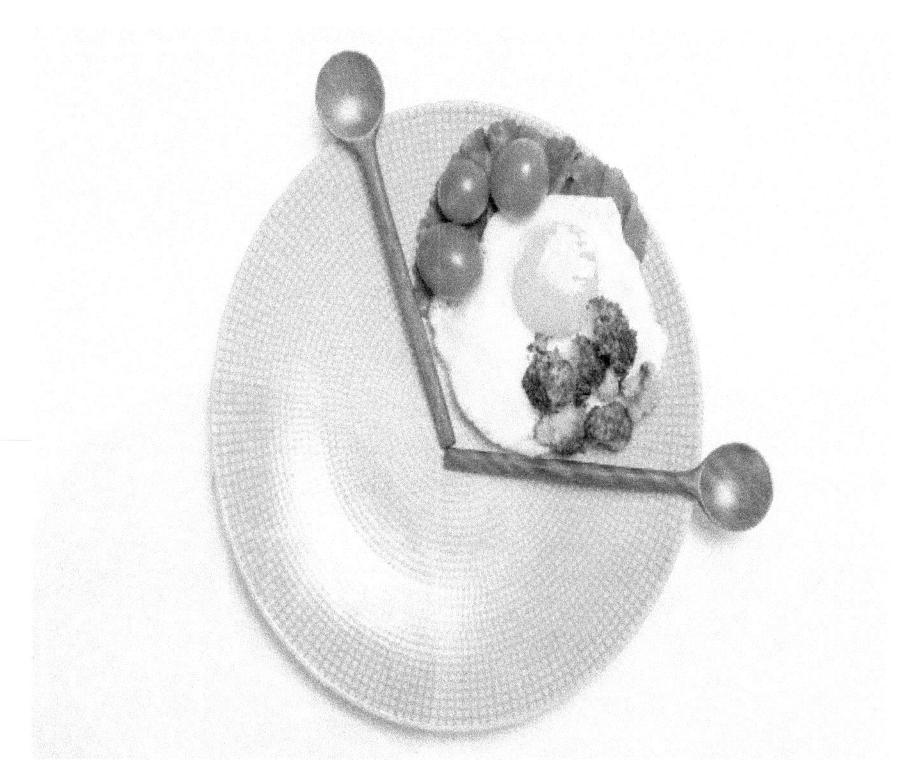

Chapter 2: The 16/8 Method

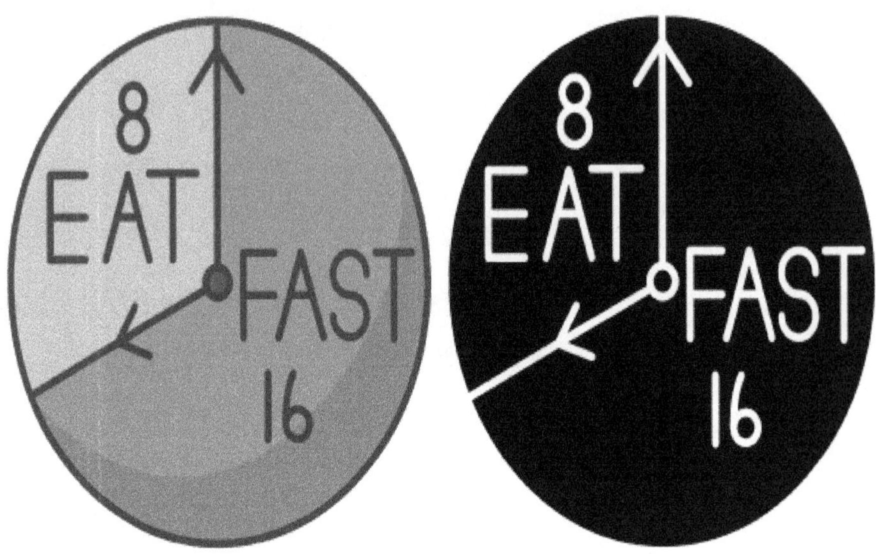

The 16/8 method is one of the most popular forms of intermittent fasting. It involves fasting for 16 hours and eating during an 8 hour window. This method is also known as the Leangains method, named after its creator, Martin Berkhan. In this chapter, we will explore the 16/8 method in more detail and discuss how to implement it into your daily routine.

1. How the 16/8 Method Works:

The 16/8 method works by limiting the time during which food is consumed, giving the body a break from digestion and allowing it to shift into a state of repair and rejuvenation. During the fasting period, the body shifts into a state of ketosis, where it begins to burn stored fat for energy instead of glucose. This results in weight loss and improved metabolic health.

2. Pros and Cons of the 16/8 Method:

The 16/8 method has many potential benefits, including weight loss, improved insulin sensitivity, and a reduction in the risk of chronic diseases such as type 2 diabetes and heart disease. However, there are also potential drawbacks to consider, such as the risk of overeating during the eating window, and the potential for nutrient deficiencies if the diet is not well-planned.

3. Tips for Success with the 16/8 Method:

To achieve success with the 16/8 method, it's important to be consistent with the fasting and eating schedule, to focus on nutrient-dense foods during the eating window, and to stay hydrated during the fasting period. It's also important to be mindful of portion sizes and to listen to your body's hunger cues. Regular exercise is also important for overall health and can help to reduce feelings of hunger.

4. The 16 Hour Fast:

The first step in the 16/8 method is to fast for 16 hours. This can be done by skipping breakfast and eating your first meal at lunchtime, or by having an early dinner and skipping breakfast the next day. The key is to find a fasting schedule that works for you and your lifestyle.

5. The 8 Hour Eating Window:

After the 16 hour fast, you have an 8 hour window during which you can eat. During this time, you should focus on nutrient-dense foods, such as fruits, vegetables, lean proteins, and whole grains. Avoid processed foods and sugary drinks.

6. Timing of Meals:

The timing of your meals is important for the 16/8 method to be effective. It's best to have your last meal at least 2-3 hours before bed to give your body enough time to digest before you enter your fasting period.

7. Hydration:

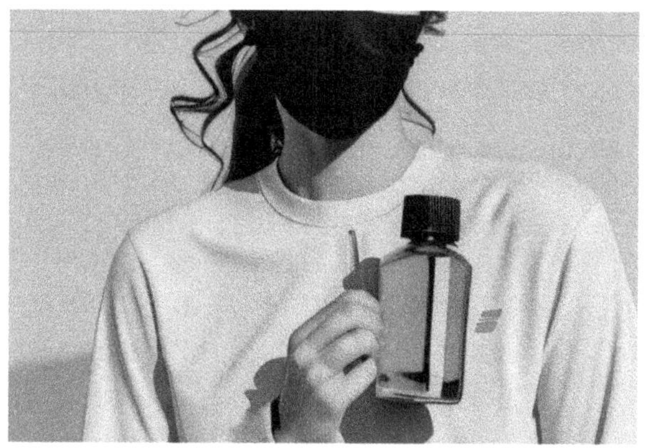

It's important to stay hydrated during the fasting period, especially if you're feeling thirsty. Drinking water, herbal tea, or coffee (without added sugar) during the fasting period is allowed.

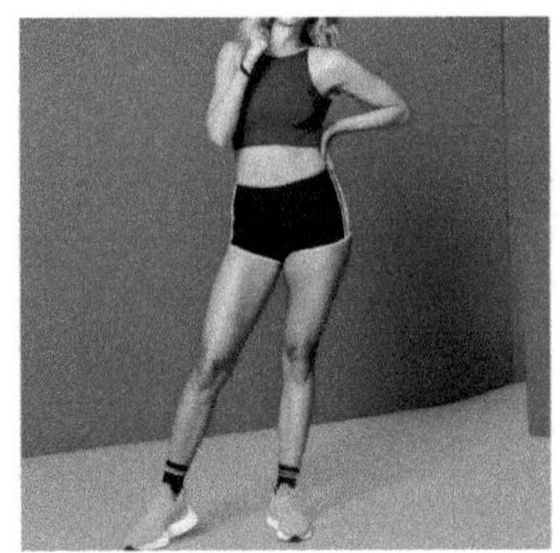

8. Exercise:

Regular exercise is an important component of a healthy lifestyle, and it's especially important during intermittent fasting. Exercise can help you stay energized and reduce feelings of hunger.

9. Flexibility:

It's important to remember that the 16/8 method is flexible, and you can adjust the timing of your fasting and eating periods to suit your schedule and lifestyle.

It's also important to remember that the 16/8 method is not suitable for everyone, and it's best to consult with a healthcare professional before starting any new diet or exercise regimen.

In conclusion, the 16/8 method is a popular form of intermittent fasting that involves fasting for 16 hours and eating during an 8 hour window. It's important to find a fasting schedule that works for you, to focus on nutrient-dense foods during the eating window, and to stay hydrated during the fasting period. Regular exercise and flexibility with timing is also important. Remember that it's a lifestyle change that requires commitment and consistency to achieve your goals.

Remember to consult with a healthcare professional before starting any new diet or exercise regimen.

Chapter 3: The 5:2 Diet

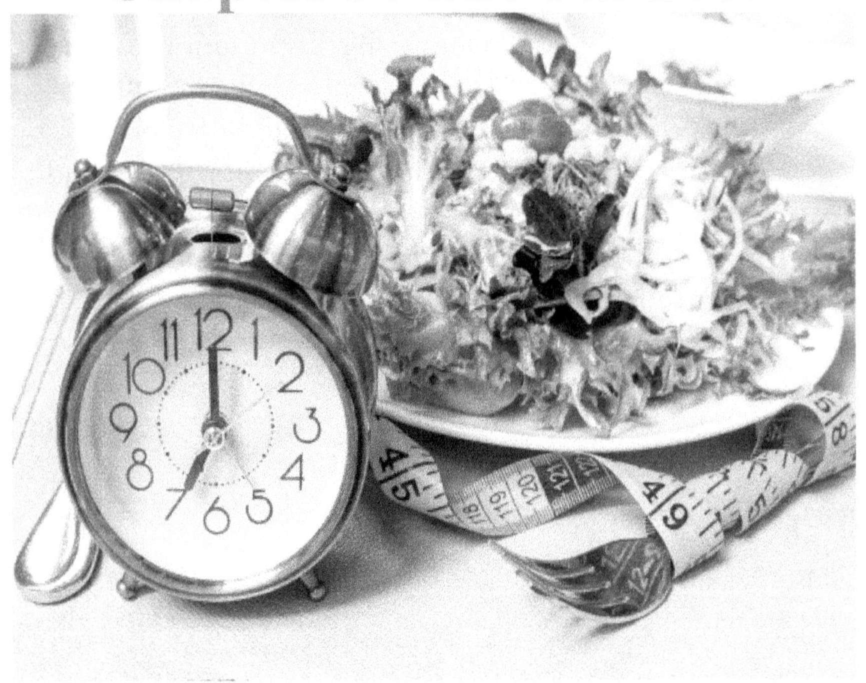

The 5:2 diet is a form of intermittent fasting that involves eating normally for five days a week and restricting calories to a very low level for the other two days. In this chapter, we will explore the science behind the 5:2 diet, the potential benefits and drawbacks of this method, and tips for success.

1. **How the 5:2 Diet Works:**

The 5:2 diet works by creating a calorie deficit over the course of the week by limiting calorie intake for two non-consecutive days. This calorie deficit is thought to result in weight loss and improved metabolic health. The two days of calorie restriction should be non-consecutive, and the calorie intake should be limited to around 500-600 calories for women and 600-800 calories for men.

2. Pros and Cons of the 5:2 Diet:

The 5:2 diet has many potential benefits, including weight loss, improved insulin sensitivity, and a reduction in the risk of chronic diseases such as type 2 diabetes and heart disease. However, there are also potential drawbacks to consider, such as the risk of overeating during the non-restricted days, and the potential for nutrient deficiencies if the diet is not well-planned.

3. Tips for Success with the 5:2 Diet:

To achieve success with the 5:2 diet, it's important to be consistent with the fasting and eating schedule, to focus on nutrient-dense foods during the non-restricted days, and to stay hydrated during the restricted days. It's also important to be mindful of portion sizes and to listen to your body's hunger cues. Regular exercise is also important for overall health and can help to reduce feelings of hunger.

It's also important to remember that the 5:2 diet is not suitable for everyone, and it's best to consult with a healthcare professional before starting any new diet or exercise regimen.

In conclusion, the 5:2 diet is a form of intermittent fasting that involves eating normally for five days a week and restricting calories to a very low level for the other two days. It has many potential benefits, but it's important to be mindful of the potential drawbacks and to listen to your body's hunger cues. Regular exercise and consistency with fasting and eating schedule are key to success with the 5:2 diet. Remember to consult with a healthcare professional before starting any new diet or exercise regimen.

Chapter 4: The Alternate Day Fasting

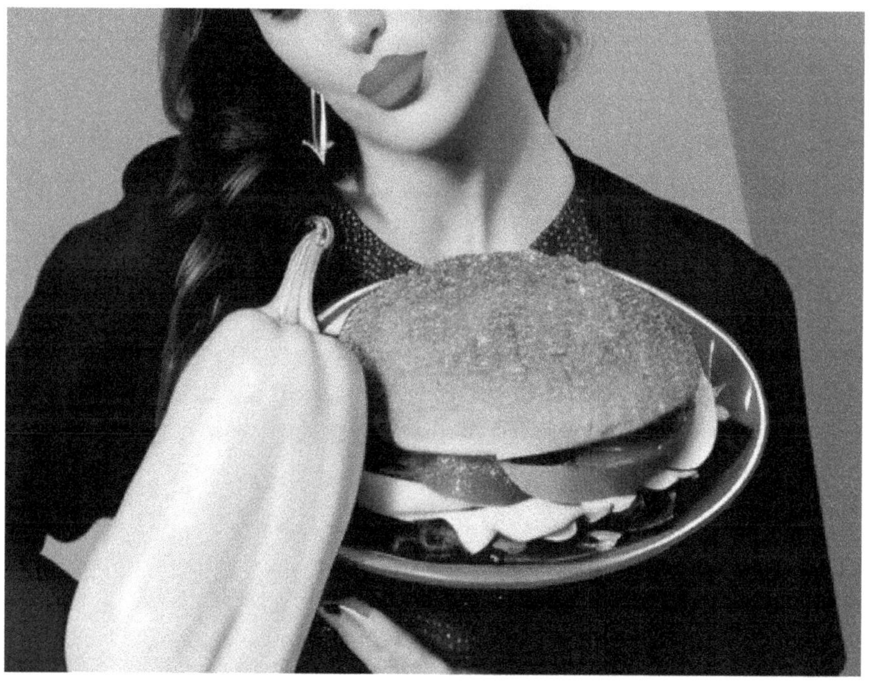

The Alternate Day Fasting (ADF) is a form of intermittent fasting that involves alternating between days of calorie restriction and days of normal eating. This chapter will explore the science behind ADF, the potential benefits and drawbacks of this method, and tips for success.

1. **How the Alternate Day Fasting Works:**

The ADF method works by alternating between days of calorie restriction, typically consuming around 20-25% of the usual calorie intake, and days of normal eating. The idea behind this method is that the body will enter a state of "metabolic switching" on the restricted days, leading to improved insulin sensitivity and weight loss.

2. Pros and Cons of the Alternate Day Fasting:

The ADF method has been shown to result in weight loss, improved insulin sensitivity, and a reduction in the risk of chronic diseases such as type 2 diabetes and heart disease. However, it can be difficult to stick to the restricted days and can result in feelings of deprivation, which may lead to overeating on the non-restricted days. Additionally, ADF may be a more challenging method for those with a history of disordered eating.

3. Tips for Success with the Alternate Day Fasting:

To achieve success with the ADF method, it's important to be consistent with the fasting and eating schedule, to focus on nutrient-dense foods during the non-restricted days, and to stay hydrated during the restricted days. It's also important to listen to your body's hunger cues and to be mindful of portion sizes. Regular exercise is also important for overall health and can help to reduce feelings of hunger.

In conclusion, Alternate Day Fasting (ADF) is a form of intermittent fasting that involves alternating between days of calorie restriction and days of normal eating. It has many potential benefits, but it's important to be mindful of the potential drawbacks and to listen to your body's hunger cues. Regular exercise and consistency with fasting and eating schedules are key to success with ADF. Remember to consult with a healthcare professional before starting any new diet or exercise regimen.

Chapter 5: Combining Intermittent Fasting with Exercise

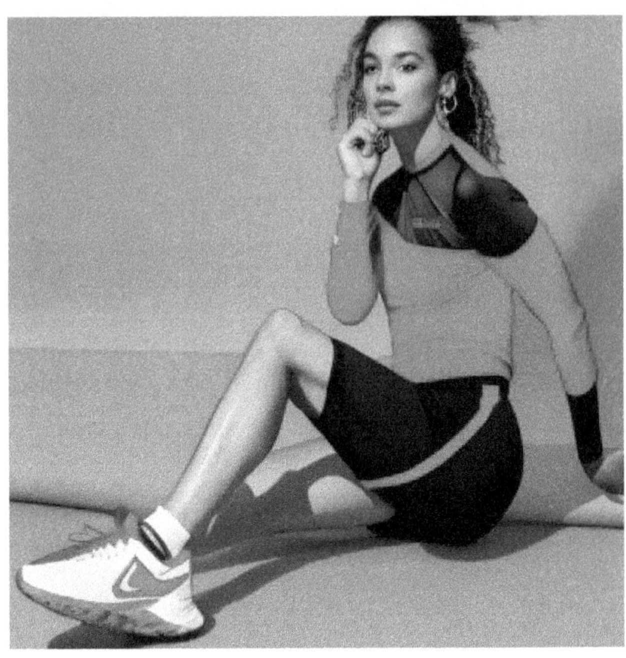

Intermittent fasting and exercise are two powerful tools for improving overall health and fitness. This chapter will explore the benefits of combining these two practices, as well as tips for making the most of your workout while fasting.

1. **The Benefits of Combining Intermittent Fasting with Exercise:**

Intermittent fasting and exercise both have their own set of benefits, such as weight loss, improved insulin sensitivity, and increased muscle mass. When combined, they can amplify each other's effects, resulting in even greater improvements in overall health and fitness. Additionally, fasting before exercise can improve endurance, increase the release of growth hormone, and improve fat burning during the workout.

2. **Best Types of Exercise for Intermittent Fasting:**

Low-intensity exercises such as yoga, light cardio, and steady-state cardio are ideal for intermittent fasting as they do not require a lot of energy and do not increase appetite as much as high-intensity exercises. High-intensity interval training (HIIT) and weightlifting can be done during the eating window but it is important to listen to your body and to stop exercising if you feel weak or dizzy.

3. **Tips for Exercising While Fasting:**

To get the most out of your workout while fasting, it's important to stay hydrated and to focus on low-intensity exercises such as yoga or light cardio. Avoiding high-intensity workouts, such as weightlifting, during fasting periods is recommended as it requires more energy and may be challenging. It's also important to listen to your body and to stop exercising if you feel weak or dizzy.

4. **Post-Workout Nutrition:**

After a workout, it's important to replenish your energy stores by consuming a meal or a snack that includes carbohydrates and protein. This will help to repair muscle tissue, boost recovery and prevent muscle breakdown.

In conclusion, combining intermittent fasting with exercise can enhance the benefits of both practices and lead to greater improvements in overall health and fitness. It's important to stay hydrated and focus on low-intensity exercises while fasting, and to consume a meal or snack that includes carbohydrates and protein after a workout to boost recovery and prevent muscle breakdown. Remember to listen to your body and to stop exercising if you feel weak or dizzy.

Chapter 6: Intermittent Fasting and Weight Loss

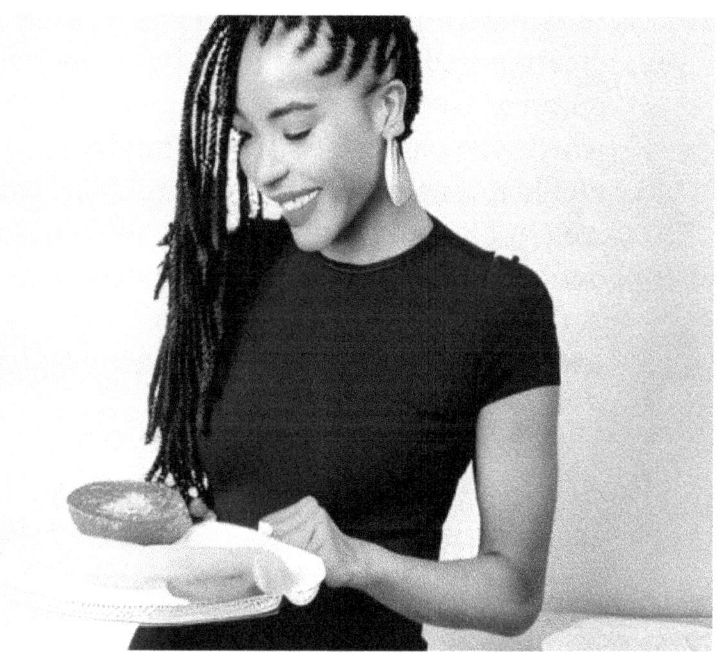

Intermittent fasting is a popular weight loss strategy that involves alternating periods of eating and fasting. This chapter will explore how intermittent fasting can help with weight loss, the factors that affect weight loss with intermittent fasting, and tips for maintaining weight loss with intermittent fasting.

1. **How Intermittent Fasting Can Help with Weight Loss:**

Intermittent fasting can help with weight loss by creating a calorie deficit and by promoting fat burning. By restricting the window of time during which you can eat, you are naturally reducing the number of calories you consume. This can lead to weight loss, particularly if you are in a calorie deficit. Additionally, during a fasted state, your body shifts from burning glucose to burning fat for energy, which can lead to increased fat burning.

2. **Factors that Affect Weight Loss with Intermittent Fasting:**

There are several factors that can affect weight loss with intermittent fasting, such as the type of intermittent fasting method you choose, your diet, and your activity level. The 16/8 method, for example, is more effective than the 5:2 diet, as it allows for more consistent calorie restriction. Additionally, a diet high in nutrient-dense, whole foods will support weight loss, while a diet high in processed foods will not. And, regular exercise can boost weight loss and improve overall health.

3. **Maintaining Weight Loss with Intermittent Fasting:**

Maintaining weight loss with intermittent fasting is possible, but it requires consistency and discipline. A key to success is sticking to a consistent eating schedule and avoiding snacking during fasting periods. It's also important to focus on nutrient-dense, whole foods during eating periods and to avoid processed and high-calorie foods. Additionally, regular exercise can help to maintain weight loss and improve overall health.

In conclusion, Intermittent fasting can be an effective weight loss strategy when combined with a calorie deficit and healthy eating habits. Factors such as the type of intermittent fasting method, diet, and activity level can affect weight loss. To maintain weight loss with intermittent fasting, consistency and discipline are key. Stick to a consistent eating schedule, limit snacking, focus on nutrient-dense foods and include regular exercise. As always, it's important to consult with a healthcare professional before starting any new weight loss program.

Chapter 7: Intermittent Fasting and Health

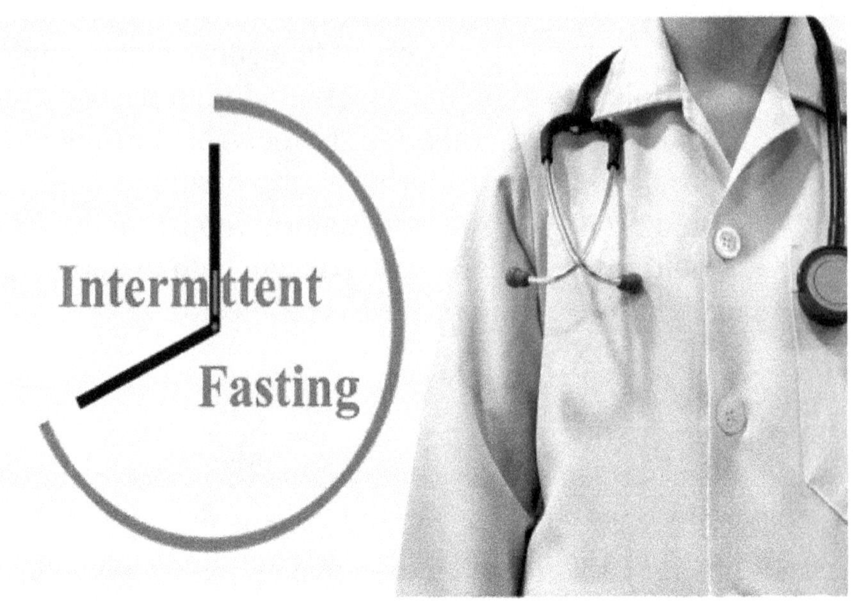

Intermittent fasting is not only a popular weight loss strategy but also has potential health benefits. This chapter will explore some of the ways in which intermittent fasting can benefit health, including the effects on metabolism, heart health, and brain function, as well as risks and precautions.

1. The Health Benefits of Intermittent Fasting:

Intermittent fasting can improve the body's metabolism by increasing insulin sensitivity and reducing inflammation. During a fasted state, the body shifts from burning glucose to burning fat for energy, which can lead to increased insulin sensitivity and improved blood sugar control. Additionally, fasting has been shown to reduce inflammation in the body, which is a risk factor for many chronic diseases.

2. Risks and Precautions of Intermittent Fasting:

Intermittent fasting can be a safe and effective weight loss strategy for most people, but it may not be suitable for everyone. People with certain medical conditions, such as diabetes, pregnant or breastfeeding women, and those who are underweight or have a history of eating disorders should consult a healthcare professional before starting intermittent fasting. Additionally, people who are taking certain medications may need to adjust their dosage or timing when fasting.

3. Intermittent Fasting and Chronic Diseases:

Intermittent fasting may have a positive effect on heart health by reducing blood pressure and improving cholesterol levels. Studies have found that intermittent fasting can lower blood pressure and improve the ratio of "good" HDL cholesterol to "bad" LDL cholesterol. Additionally, intermittent fasting may help to reduce the risk of certain chronic diseases such as type 2 diabetes, cancer and Alzheimer's disease.

4. Brain Function:

Intermittent fasting may also have benefits for brain function by increasing the production of brain-derived neurotrophic factor (BDNF), a protein that promotes the growth and survival of nerve cells. This can lead to improved memory and cognitive function.

It's important to note that while there is promising research on the potential health benefits of intermittent fasting, more studies are needed to fully understand the effects and to determine the long-term safety. Additionally, it is important to consult with a healthcare professional before starting any new diet or exercise program, particularly if you have any health conditions or concerns.

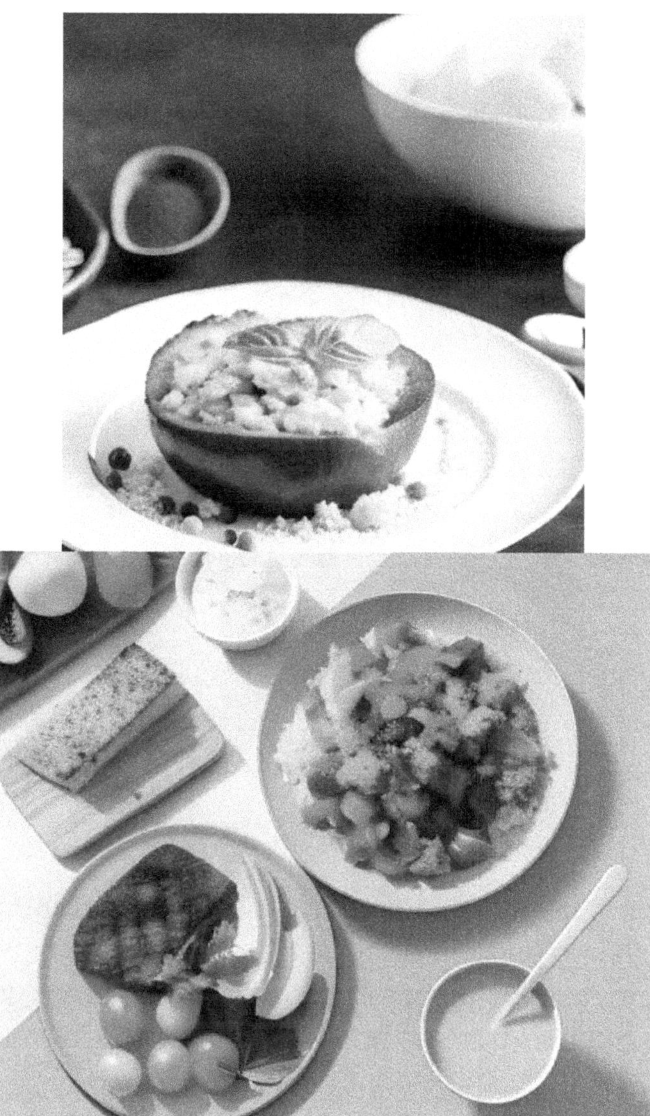

Chapter 8: Breaking a Fast

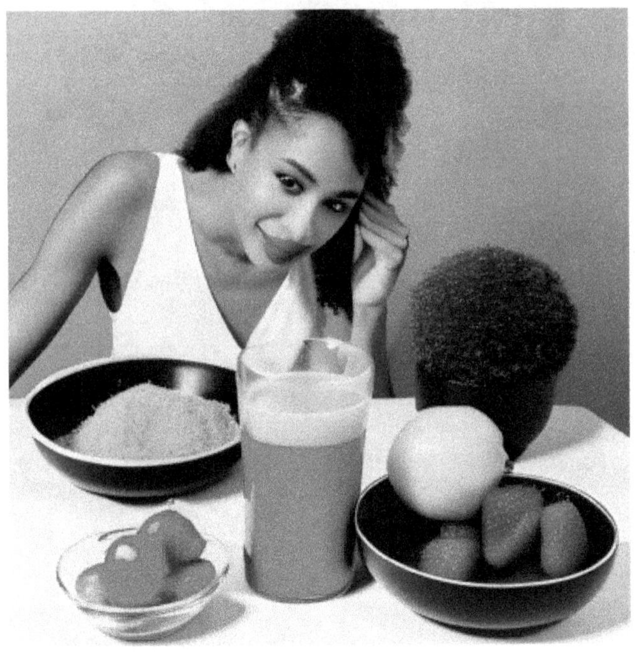

Breaking a fast is an important aspect of intermittent fasting. It's important to break a fast in a way that is safe and supports the benefits of the fast. This chapter will explore the best ways to break a fast and tips for making the transition back to eating.

1. How to Safely Break a Fast:

After a period of fasting, the body may be in a state of heightened insulin sensitivity. It's important to ease into eating by starting with small, nutrient-dense meals and gradually increasing portion sizes. Avoid consuming large amounts of processed or high-carbohydrate foods as it may cause a spike in blood sugar levels. Additionally, it's important to pay attention to how your body is feeling and to stop eating if you start to feel unwell.

2. What to Eat After a Fast:

The best foods to eat after a fast are nutrient-dense, high in protein, and easy to digest. These include fruits and vegetables, lean protein sources, such as fish or chicken, and healthy fats, such as avocado or nuts. Whole grains and legumes can also be included, but it's important to start with small portions to see how your body reacts.

3. Tips for a Smooth Transition:

One of the best ways to make the transition back to eating after a fast is to focus on simple, whole foods. Avoid processed foods, sugary drinks, and excessive caffeine. It's also important to stay hydrated, as dehydration is common during fasting, so drink plenty of water and other fluids during the breaking of fast.

4. Listen to your body:

Breaking a fast is a personal process and it's important to listen to your body and adjust your eating habits as needed. Some people may feel comfortable breaking a fast with a large meal, while others may prefer a more gradual approach.

5. Avoid snacking:

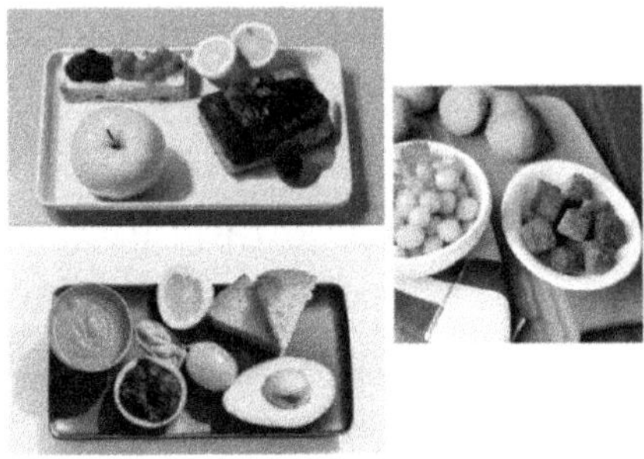

To break the fast and avoid snacking between meals, it's important to plan your meals and eat at regular intervals. Avoiding snacking between meals and consuming large meals will help to regulate blood sugar levels and prevent overeating.

It's important to note that everyone's body is different, and what works for one person may not work for another. It's important to pay attention to how your body reacts to breaking a fast and adjust your approach as needed.

Additionally, it's important to consult with a healthcare professional before starting any new diet or exercise program, particularly if you have any health conditions or concerns.

Conclusion

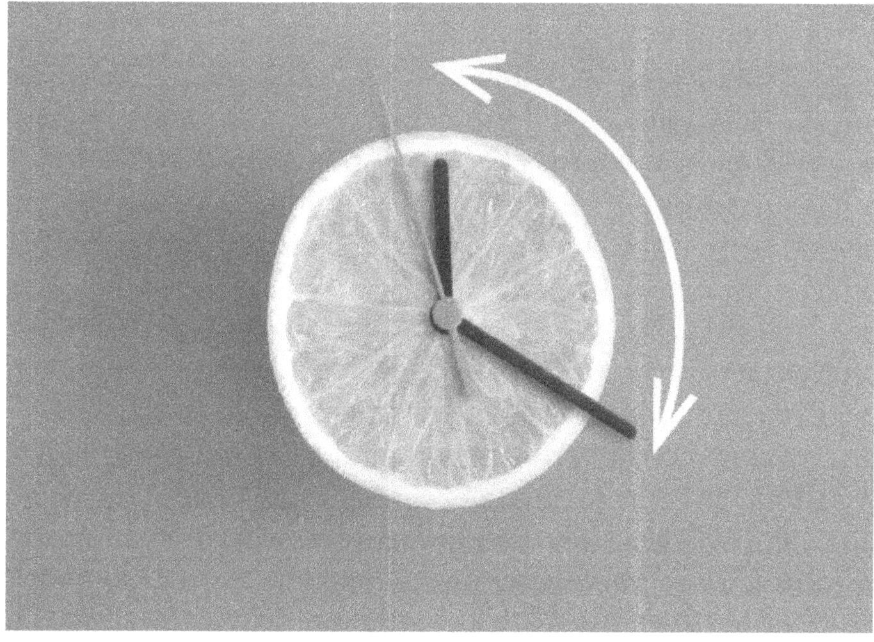

Intermittent fasting has been shown to have a number of health benefits and can be an effective tool for weight loss. However, it is important to remember that it is not a one-size-fits-all approach and may not be suitable for everyone. It is always recommended to consult with a healthcare professional before starting any new diet or exercise regimen.

Final thoughts on intermittent fasting include the importance of listening to your body's hunger cues, starting slowly and gradually increasing the frequency and duration of your fasts, and being consistent with your chosen method. It is also important to remember that intermittent fasting should be used in combination with a healthy diet and regular exercise for optimal results.

Frequently Asked Questions:

1. Can I have coffee or tea while fasting?
2. Can I exercise while fasting?
3. How long should I fast for?
4. Can I eat whatever I want during my eating window?
5. Is it okay to break a fast with a large meal?

Resources for further learning include books, websites, and online communities dedicated to intermittent fasting and its various methods. It is important to seek out accurate and reliable information to ensure that you are following a safe and effective plan. Additionally, consulting with a healthcare professional or registered dietitian can provide personalized advice and support.